Prevention Is the Best Medicine

For Parents and Elected Officials

By Alfred Brock

Contents

Introduction 5

Chapter 1 - Dangers of Illicit Drugs to Teenagers 7

Chapter 2 – Drugs Are Not A Recreational Activity...................10

Chapter 3 – Profits in the Illicit Drug Markets 14

Chapter 4 – Alcohol 16

Chapter 5 – Ayahuasca 19

Chapter 6 - Cannabis (Marijuana/Pot/Weed).........................22

Chapter 7 - Central Nervous System Depressants (Benzos) 25

Chapter 8 - Cocaine (Coke/Crack)......................................29

Chapter 9 – GHB 32

Chapter 10 – Hallucinogens 35

Chapter 11 – Heroin..38

Chapter 12 – Inhalants...41

Chapter 13 – Ketamine 44

Chapter 14 – Khat 47

Chapter 15 – Kratom...50

Chapter 16 - LSD (Acid) 53

Chapter 17 - MDMA (Ecstasy/Molly) 56

Chapter 18 - Mescaline (Peyote) 59

Chapter 19 - Methamphetamine (Crystal/Meth) 62

Chapter 20 - Over-the-Counter Medicines—Dextromethorphan (DXM)..65

Chapter 21 - Over-the-Counter Medicines—Loperamide 68

Chapter 22 - PCP (Angel Dust) 71

Chapter 23 - Prescription Opioids (Oxy/Percs) 74

Chapter 24 - Prescription Stimulants (Speed)............................77

Chapter 25 - Psilocybin (Magic Mushrooms/Shrooms) 81

Chapter 26 - Rohypnol® (Flunitrazepam/Roofies) 84

Chapter 27 – Salvia 87

Chapter 28 - Steroids (Anabolic)...90

Chapter 29 - Synthetic Cannabinoids (K2/Spice) 93

Chapter 30 - Synthetic Cathinones (Bath Salts/Flakka) 97

Chapter 31 - Tobacco/Nicotine and Vaping.............................100

Chapter 32 – Prevention 103

What is Prevention? 103

How Does One Go About Starting A Drug Use Prevention
Program for Children and Teenagers? 106

Principles of Drug Addiction Treatment – From NIDA (National
Institute on Drug Abuse)..110

INDEX OF SUPPORT MATERIALS 114

Introduction

Too often in my work involving teenagers, young adults, older adults and even seniors, I find a general lack of basic information. Because of this dearth of information about the impacts that drugs have on their lives, livelihoods and futures they often find themselves in a world of woe that they never imagined. Time, and more importantly, lives are being wasted because these things are not discussed openly.

How can this be corrected? The romanticization of drug use and the black market businesses associated with them needs to be updated. One can find many 'entertainment' vehicles in movies, music and other mediums that elevate the needless suffering and personal problems caused by drug use to heroic levels. Recent reports from the entertainment industry make it clear that this material is not about drug use it is being created by people who use the drugs. Their careers are built on a de facto advertising industry that supports the manufacturing, marketing, distribution and sales of the drugs they include in their materials.

This book is intended to allow parents and elected officials to become aware of the basic information they need to know about what is going on in our communities. It is important for parents because even when schools may be experiencing high levels of drug use and all the problems associated with drug use the information may never reach the parents. This is unfortunate for the children forced to attend these schools. Growing up is hard to do. Growing up in the presence of the violence and mental illness that comes along with illicit drug use is a burden children should not have to bear.

Elected Officials should be aware of these drugs so they can be prepared to listen to and work with concerned parents and children in their sphere of influence. Elected Officials, because of the nature of the tax system in the United States, can weigh in on issues faced by local schools. It is unfortunate that as local school boards fight over whether or not allow books about drugs and the problems they bring in the school library they are spending enormous amounts of money on 'Vape Detectors' and security devices. Obviously there are plenty of problems involving the schools.

This book provides a baseline of information that can provide a parent or elected official enough information to recognize the problems around them.

It is clear at this point that four things can be stated :

1. We cannot arrest our way out of this drug problem
2. Children and Adolescents should not use drugs
3. Taking Drugs is not a Recreational Activity
4. Prevention is successful and necessary

Chapter 1 - Dangers of Illicit Drugs to Teenagers

Illicit drug use among teenagers poses a range of physical, mental, and social dangers that can have lasting negative impacts on their health and well-being. Here are some of the key dangers associated with illicit drug use among teenagers:

Physical Health Risks:

Addiction: Adolescents' brains are still developing, and they are more susceptible to developing addiction than adults. Early drug use can increase the risk of developing a substance use disorder later in life.

Overdose: Teenagers may underestimate the potency and potential dangers of drugs, leading to accidental overdose, which can be fatal.

Health Problems: Illicit drugs can have detrimental effects on physical health, including heart problems, respiratory issues, liver damage, and compromised immune systems.

Mental Health Risks:

Mental Illness: Drug use during adolescence can increase the risk of developing mental health disorders such as anxiety, depression, and psychosis. It can also exacerbate existing mental health issues.

Cognitive Impairment: Drug use can negatively impact cognitive functions like memory, attention, and decision-making, which can hinder academic and personal development.

Social Consequences:

School Performance: Substance abuse can lead to poor school performance, absenteeism, and dropping out, which can limit future educational and career opportunities.

Relationships: Drug use can strain relationships with family, friends, and peers. Teens might engage in risky behaviors that lead to conflicts and alienation.

Legal Issues: Illicit drug use is against the law, and teenagers caught using or possessing drugs can face legal consequences that affect their future prospects.

Risky Behavior:

Impaired Judgment: Drugs can impair decision-making and increase the likelihood of engaging in risky behaviors, such as unsafe sex or driving under the influence.

Accidents and Injuries: Impaired coordination and perception caused by drug use can increase the risk of accidents, injuries, and even fatalities.

Gateway to Further Drug Use:

Progression: Using one illicit substance can make teenagers more susceptible to trying other, potentially more dangerous, drugs. This can lead to a cycle of experimentation and increased risk.

Long-Term Consequences:

Brain Development: Adolescence is a critical period for brain development. Drug use during this time can disrupt normal brain development and have lasting effects on cognitive abilities and emotional regulation.

Interference with Future Goals: Continued drug use can limit teenagers' potential by affecting their ability to pursue education, careers, and personal goals.

Hidden Dangers:

Laced or Contaminated Drugs: Illicit drugs are often not regulated, and teenagers might unknowingly consume substances laced with dangerous additives or contaminants that can lead to severe health complications.

Preventing illicit drug use among teenagers requires a multi-faceted approach involving education, open communication, supportive environments, and access to mental health resources. Parents, schools, communities, and healthcare professionals all play crucial roles in addressing these dangers and providing teenagers with the tools they need to make informed and healthy choices.

Chapter 2 – Drugs Are Not A Recreational Activity

Trivializing the Dangers of Drug Use: Societal Problems Arising from Referring to Drug Use as a Recreational Activity

In recent years, a concerning trend has emerged within society — the trivialization of drug use by labeling it as a recreational activity. This normalization of drug use has far-reaching consequences that extend beyond individual choices to impact entire communities and societies. While recreational drug use might appear harmless on the surface, its implications are much more complex and multifaceted. This essay delves into the problems associated with downplaying the dangers of drug use and framing it as a mere recreational pursuit. From health risks to social implications, this trend has the potential to erode the fabric of society and jeopardize the well-being of future generations.

I. Health Risks and Public Health Concerns:

Underestimation of Harm: Referring to drug use as recreational downplays the serious health risks and consequences associated with substance abuse. By using this terminology, society can unwittingly send the message that drug use is a benign activity, leading to a lack of awareness regarding potential harm.

Healthcare Burden: Trivializing drug use may contribute to a strain on healthcare systems, as individuals engaging in recreational drug use may not seek medical assistance promptly, fearing social judgment or failing to recognize the severity of their condition.

Overlooking Addiction: Using recreational language for drug use can divert attention from the potential for addiction. This can prevent individuals from recognizing signs of addiction early, delaying interventions and exacerbating the problem.

II. Undermining Anti-Drug Initiatives:

Mixed Messaging: Presenting drug use as recreational undermines anti-drug campaigns and education efforts, creating a contradictory narrative that weakens the effectiveness of prevention programs.

Youth Influence: By portraying drug use as recreational, society inadvertently makes drug use more appealing to impressionable youth, contributing to increased experimentation and potential addiction in younger generations.

Lax Attitudes: Normalizing drug use by referring to it as recreational can lead to attitudes of complacency, making it harder to rally public support for policies aimed at reducing drug-related harm.

III. Societal Breakdown and Fragmentation:

Erosion of Social Fabric: Trivializing the dangers of drug use can contribute to a weakening of community bonds, as recreational drug use may be seen as an individual right rather than a collective responsibility.

Isolation and Stigmatization: People struggling with drug addiction might be less likely to seek help due to societal attitudes that dismiss their challenges. Trivializing drug use perpetuates a stigma that isolates those in need of assistance.

Family Disintegration: The normalization of recreational drug use can strain family relationships as individuals may prioritize their addiction over familial responsibilities, leading to broken homes and strained parent-child relationships.

IV. Economic and Legal Consequences:

Lost Productivity: The impact of drug use on the workforce cannot be overlooked. By treating drug use as recreational, society may underestimate its economic toll due to decreased productivity and increased absenteeism.

Legal Implications: Downplaying the dangers of drug use may lead to a perception that drug-related crimes are less serious. This could weaken law enforcement efforts and undermine the justice system's ability to deter illicit drug activities.

V. International Ramifications:

Global Drug Trade: Trivializing drug use can inadvertently fuel the international drug trade, as demand remains strong due to the perception of drugs as recreational rather than harmful.

Social Inequities: Developing countries with limited resources for addiction treatment may suffer disproportionately from the consequences of trivializing drug use. The impact of addiction on vulnerable populations could worsen due to reduced global attention.

Therefore the trivialization of drug use by framing it as a recreational activity poses a multitude of problems for society at large. From jeopardizing public health to undermining anti-drug initiatives and contributing to societal breakdown, the consequences are wide-ranging and profound. It is imperative that society acknowledges and addresses the dangers of such a perspective, promoting awareness, education, and empathy. By understanding the gravity of the issue and reframing the conversation around drug use, we can collectively work toward a healthier, safer, and more cohesive society.

Estimating the profits realized by drug dealers in the United States is challenging due to the illicit and underground nature of the drug trade. Additionally, profits can vary significantly based on factors such as the type of drug, location, distribution network, and market demand. However, I can provide you with some rough figures based on historical data and expert estimates as of my last knowledge update in September 2021.

Cocaine: The cocaine market in the United States is estimated to be worth billions of dollars annually. In the 2010s, it was estimated that a kilogram of cocaine could be purchased for around $12,000 to $15,000 wholesale and could be sold on the street for $30,000 to $40,000 or more. With multiple transactions along the distribution chain, profits can accumulate substantially.

Heroin: Heroin profits can also be substantial due to the high demand for the drug. Estimates suggest that a kilogram of heroin could be purchased for around $60,000 to $80,000 wholesale and sold for significantly higher prices on the street.

Marijuana: The marijuana market is significant in the United States due to its widespread use and changing legal landscape. Estimates vary, but the wholesale price of a pound of marijuana could range from a few hundred dollars to over $2,000, depending on factors like quality and location. Retail prices are considerably higher, potentially generating substantial profits.

Methamphetamine: The methamphetamine market has been a concern due to its impact on communities. Wholesale prices for a pound of methamphetamine could range from a few thousand dollars to over $10,000, with street prices being considerably higher.

Synthetic Drugs: The profits from synthetic drugs like synthetic opioids and designer drugs can also be significant, especially when considering the potential for strong demand and the low cost of production for some synthetic substances.

It's important to note that these figures are very rough estimates and can vary widely based on market conditions, law enforcement efforts, changes in drug purity, and other factors. Additionally, the illegal drug trade has likely evolved since my last update, and new trends and pricing dynamics may have emerged.

The profits realized by drug dealers are ultimately driven by the interplay of supply and demand, law enforcement efforts, and the risks associated with participating in the illicit drug trade. It's also crucial to emphasize that these profits come at a significant cost to public health, safety, and social well-being.

Chapter 4 – Alcohol

Alcohol use among children and teenagers poses a range of serious dangers to their physical, mental, and social well-being. Adolescents' bodies and brains are still developing, and alcohol can have particularly harmful effects on their growth and development. Here are some of the key dangers associated with alcohol use among children and teenagers:

Physical Health Risks:

Brain Development: Alcohol can interfere with the development of the adolescent brain, potentially leading to cognitive deficits, memory problems, and impaired decision-making abilities.

Physical Health Issues: Teenagers who drink alcohol are more prone to accidents, injuries, and risky behaviors due to impaired coordination, reflexes, and judgment. Alcohol use can also contribute to liver damage, heart problems, and compromised immune systems.

Mental Health Risks:

Depression and Anxiety: Alcohol use during adolescence can increase the risk of developing mental health disorders like depression and anxiety. It can also exacerbate existing mental health issues.

Suicidal Behavior: Alcohol use is associated with a higher risk of suicidal thoughts and attempts among teenagers, possibly due to the depressant effects of alcohol on mood and judgment.

Academic and Social Consequences:

Poor School Performance: Alcohol use can lead to decreased academic performance, absenteeism, and a lack of motivation, which can hinder educational and career opportunities.

Peer Pressure and Relationships: Teenagers may face peer pressure to drink, leading to potentially harmful social dynamics and compromised relationships. Alcohol-related behaviors can also strain friendships and family relationships.

Risk of Addiction:

Vulnerability to Addiction: Adolescent brains are more susceptible to addiction, and early alcohol use increases the risk of developing alcohol use disorder or other substance use disorders later in life.

Gateway to Further Substance Use: Alcohol use can serve as a gateway to experimenting with other substances, which can lead to more serious substance abuse problems.

Legal Consequences:

Underage Drinking Laws: Drinking alcohol is illegal for individuals under the legal drinking age. Teenagers caught consuming alcohol can face legal consequences, including fines, suspension of driver's licenses, and other legal penalties.

Impaired Decision-Making:

Risky Behaviors: Alcohol impairs judgment and decision-making, leading to risky behaviors such as unprotected sex, driving under the influence, and involvement in accidents.

Long-Term Effects:

Memory and Learning Impairment: Excessive alcohol use during adolescence can lead to long-term deficits in memory, attention, and learning abilities.

Behavioral Problems: Teenagers who engage in alcohol use are more likely to exhibit behavioral problems and engage in delinquent or criminal activities.

Preventing alcohol use among children and teenagers requires a combination of parental guidance, education, and community support. Open communication about the dangers of alcohol, setting clear expectations, and providing alternatives to risky behaviors are crucial strategies for reducing the negative impact of alcohol on young individuals. Additionally, involving schools, healthcare professionals, and community organizations in prevention efforts can help create an environment that supports healthy choices and discourages underage drinking.

Chapter 5 – Ayahuasca

Ayahuasca is a powerful hallucinogenic brew traditionally used in indigenous Amazonian rituals for spiritual and healing purposes. While some proponents claim potential therapeutic benefits, it is important to note that Ayahuasca is not without risks, especially for children and teenagers. Due to the lack of comprehensive research and the potential for serious physical, mental, and emotional side effects, Ayahuasca use among this age group is generally not recommended. Here are some of the dangers associated with Ayahuasca use for children and teenagers:

Brain Development: Adolescence is a critical period of brain development. Introducing psychoactive substances like Ayahuasca during this time can interfere with the natural maturation of the brain, potentially leading to long-lasting cognitive and emotional effects.

Psychological Risks:

Psychological Vulnerability: Adolescents' minds are still developing, and they are more susceptible to psychological distress. Ayahuasca's intense and unpredictable effects could exacerbate or trigger mental health issues such as anxiety, depression, or psychosis.

Hallucinogenic Effects: Ayahuasca can induce hallucinations and altered states of consciousness that might be overwhelming and confusing for young individuals. These experiences can be distressing and potentially traumatizing, particularly if the user lacks proper preparation and guidance.

Physical Risks:

Physical Health: Ayahuasca can cause physical discomfort, vomiting, diarrhea, and dehydration. Children and teenagers may be more vulnerable to these adverse effects due to their developing bodies.

Lack of Regulation and Quality Control:

Potency and Dosage: Ayahuasca's potency can vary widely based on the plants used, preparation methods, and dosage. Adolescents might be at greater risk of unpredictable reactions and adverse effects due to their lower body weight and size.

Inadequate Understanding:

Maturity and Understanding: Adolescents might lack the emotional and cognitive maturity required to fully understand and process the complex and potentially overwhelming experiences induced by Ayahuasca. They might struggle to integrate these experiences into their sense of self and worldview.

Social and Ethical Concerns:

Cultural Appropriation: Ayahuasca use is deeply rooted in indigenous traditions. Exploiting or appropriating these practices without proper understanding and respect can lead to cultural insensitivity and disrespect.

Legal Implications:

Legality: Ayahuasca contains controlled substances, such as DMT (dimethyltryptamine), that are illegal in many countries. Adolescents using Ayahuasca could face legal consequences, potentially impacting their future opportunities.

Lack of Research:

Limited Data: There is limited scientific research on the safety and potential risks of Ayahuasca use in general, and even less specifically regarding its effects on adolescents. This lack of data makes it difficult to fully understand the potential risks and benefits.

Given these potential dangers, it is strongly recommended that children and teenagers avoid using Ayahuasca. If individuals are seeking therapeutic experiences or personal growth, it's advisable to pursue evidence-based therapies and approaches under the guidance of qualified mental health professionals. Adolescents' well-being and development are best supported through healthy lifestyles, proper nutrition, positive relationships, and access to appropriate medical and psychological care.

Chapter 6 - Cannabis (Marijuana/Pot/Weed)

Cannabis, commonly known as marijuana, pot, or weed, is a psychoactive drug that can have various effects on the body and mind. While some proponents argue for its medicinal uses, using cannabis during childhood and adolescence can pose several risks and dangers due to the ongoing development of the brain and body. Here are some of the key dangers associated with cannabis use among children and teenagers:

Impact on Brain Development:

Adolescence is a crucial period of brain development, and cannabis use can interfere with normal cognitive and emotional development. It can impair memory, attention, and decision-making skills, potentially affecting academic and social functioning.

Mental Health Risks:

Adolescents using cannabis are at an increased risk of developing mental health issues such as anxiety, depression, and psychosis. The risk is higher for individuals with a family history of mental health disorders.

Educational and Occupational Impact:

Cannabis use can negatively affect academic performance and educational attainment. It might limit future career opportunities if cognitive and academic abilities are compromised.

Addiction Potential:

Cannabis is not physically addictive in the same way as drugs like opioids, but it can lead to psychological dependence, especially when used regularly during adolescence.

Impaired Driving and Safety:

Cannabis use impairs motor coordination, reaction times, and judgment, which can increase the risk of accidents while driving or engaging in other potentially dangerous activities.

Gateway to Other Substances:

Some studies suggest that using cannabis during adolescence can increase the likelihood of experimenting with other, more harmful substances.

Lung Health Risks:

Smoking cannabis can harm lung health and increase the risk of respiratory problems, similar to the risks associated with smoking tobacco.

Risk of Legal Consequences:

In many places, cannabis use is illegal for individuals under a certain age. Adolescents caught using cannabis can face legal consequences that might affect their future opportunities.

Cognitive Impairment:

Regular cannabis use during adolescence can lead to long-lasting cognitive deficits, impacting memory, attention, and problem-solving skills.

Social and Relationship Impact:

Cannabis use can lead to social isolation, as young individuals might prioritize drug use over healthy relationships and social interactions.

Misinformation and Misinterpretation:

Adolescents might receive mixed messages about the safety and benefits of cannabis, leading to confusion and potentially dangerous experimentation.

Lack of Regulation and Quality Control:

Cannabis obtained from unregulated sources might be contaminated with harmful additives or have inconsistent potency, increasing the risk of negative health effects.

Preventing cannabis use among children and teenagers requires open communication, education, and creating supportive environments. Parents, schools, and community organizations play vital roles in raising awareness about the potential dangers of early cannabis use. Encouraging healthy coping mechanisms, positive self-esteem, and emotional resilience can help protect young individuals from the risks associated with cannabis use.

Chapter 7 - Central Nervous System Depressants (Benzos)

Central Nervous System (CNS) depressants, including benzodiazepines (benzos), are a class of prescription medications commonly used to treat anxiety, sleep disorders, and other conditions. However, the non-medical use of these substances, especially by children and teenagers, can have serious and potentially life-threatening consequences. Here are some of the key dangers associated with CNS depressants (benzos) use among this age group:

Respiratory Depression:

CNS depressants slow down the central nervous system, including respiratory function. Misuse or abuse of benzodiazepines can lead to respiratory depression, which can be fatal, especially in young individuals with developing respiratory systems.

Physical Health Risks:

Benzo use can lead to physical health issues such as dizziness, blurred vision, impaired coordination, and slurred speech. Adolescents might be more susceptible to these effects due to their developing bodies.

Addiction Potential:

Benzos are known to be addictive, and adolescents experimenting with these substances might be more prone to developing dependence due to their developing brain chemistry.

Mental Health Risks:

The misuse of benzodiazepines can lead to mental health issues such as increased anxiety, depression, confusion, and cognitive impairment. Young individuals might be more vulnerable to these effects.

Memory Impairment:

Benzos can impair memory and cognitive function, affecting learning and academic performance. Adolescents using these substances might struggle with memory-related tasks.

Accidents and Injuries:

CNS depressants can lead to impaired motor skills and cognitive function, increasing the risk of accidents, falls, and injuries.

Interactions with Other Substances:

Combining benzodiazepines with other substances, especially alcohol or other depressants, can amplify the depressant effects, leading to dangerous interactions and overdose.

Emotional and Behavioral Effects:

Misuse of benzodiazepines can lead to emotional instability, mood swings, and erratic behavior. Adolescents might struggle to manage their emotions while under the influence.

Withdrawal Symptoms:

Abruptly stopping benzodiazepines can lead to withdrawal symptoms, including increased anxiety, insomnia, and even seizures. Adolescents might not fully understand these potential consequences.

Risk of Overdose:

Taking high doses of benzos or combining them with other substances can lead to overdose, resulting in severe respiratory depression, unconsciousness, and even death.

Legal Consequences:

The misuse of benzodiazepines without a prescription is illegal. Adolescents caught using these substances without medical supervision can face legal repercussions.

Lack of Regulation:

Misusing benzos obtained illegally can be risky due to the lack of quality control and accurate dosage information.

Preventing the misuse of CNS depressants among children and teenagers requires education, responsible medical use, and supportive environments. Parents, healthcare providers, schools, and community organizations all play crucial roles in raising awareness about the dangers of non-medical benzo use. Encouraging healthy coping mechanisms, positive emotional well-being, and emotional resilience can help protect young individuals from the potential dangers of CNS depressant use.

Chapter 8 - Cocaine (Coke/Crack)

Cocaine, including its crystallized form known as crack cocaine, is a powerful stimulant drug that can have serious and potentially life-threatening effects, especially when used by children and teenagers. Adolescents' developing brains and bodies make them particularly vulnerable to the harmful consequences of cocaine use. Here are some of the key dangers associated with cocaine and crack cocaine use among this age group:

Cardiovascular Risks:

Cocaine use can significantly increase heart rate, blood pressure, and the risk of heart problems, including heart attacks and arrhythmias. Adolescents' cardiovascular systems are still developing, making them more susceptible to these effects.

Neurological Impact:

Cocaine can lead to neurological complications, including seizures, headaches, and strokes. Adolescents' developing brains might be particularly sensitive to these effects.

Mental Health Risks:

Cocaine use is associated with mental health issues such as anxiety, paranoia, aggression, and even mood disorders like depression. Adolescents using cocaine might be at higher risk of these negative psychological effects.

Addiction Potential:

Cocaine is highly addictive, and adolescents experimenting with the drug might be more prone to developing a substance use disorder. Early exposure to cocaine can increase the risk of long-term addiction.

Cognitive Impairment:

Cocaine use can lead to cognitive deficits, impairing memory, attention, decision-making, and problem-solving abilities. Adolescents who use cocaine might experience learning difficulties and poor academic performance.

Risky Behaviors:

Cocaine's stimulating effects can lead to risky behaviors such as reckless driving, unprotected sex, and engagement in dangerous activities.

Respiratory and Pulmonary Effects:

Cocaine use can lead to respiratory problems and lung damage. Adolescents might be more susceptible to these effects due to their developing respiratory systems.

Crack Cocaine Dangers:

Crack cocaine, a form of cocaine that is smoked, can cause intense and rapid euphoria followed by a severe "crash," leading to depression, irritability, and fatigue. The cycle of highs and lows can be particularly destabilizing for adolescents.

Financial and Legal Consequences:

Cocaine use can lead to financial strain due to the high cost of the drug. Adolescents might engage in illegal activities to obtain funds for cocaine, leading to legal consequences.

Physical Health Impact:

Cocaine use can lead to physical health issues such as weight loss, dental problems (often referred to as "cocaine teeth"), and a weakened immune system.

Lack of Regulation:

Cocaine obtained illegally is often produced and sold in unregulated environments, increasing the risk of adulteration and unpredictable potency.

Preventing cocaine and crack cocaine use among children and teenagers requires comprehensive education, open communication, and creating supportive environments. Parents, schools, and community organizations play crucial roles in raising awareness about the dangers of these substances. Fostering healthy coping mechanisms, positive self-esteem, and emotional resilience can help protect young individuals from the potential dangers of cocaine use.

Chapter 9 – GHB

GHB (gamma-hydroxybutyrate) is a central nervous system depressant that can cause sedation, euphoria, and relaxation. While it has legitimate medical uses, it is also abused as a recreational drug, which poses significant dangers to children and teenagers due to their vulnerability to its effects. Here are some of the key dangers associated with GHB use among this age group:

Physical Health Risks:

GHB is known for its depressant effects on the central nervous system. It can lead to slowed heart rate, shallow breathing, and even loss of consciousness. Adolescents' developing bodies might be more susceptible to these effects.

Overdose and Coma:

GHB has a narrow margin of safety, meaning that a small increase in dosage can lead to an overdose. Overdosing on GHB can result in a coma, which can be life-threatening and have long-term health consequences.

Memory Impairment:

GHB is notorious for causing memory loss or "blackouts." Adolescents who use GHB might not remember events that occurred while under its influence, which can have serious consequences for their safety and decision-making.

Sexual Assault and Date Rape:

GHB is sometimes referred to as the "date rape drug" due to its ability to incapacitate individuals and impair their memory. Adolescents might be particularly vulnerable to sexual assault and manipulation while under the influence of GHB.

Addiction Potential:

GHB can be addictive, leading to physical and psychological dependence. Adolescents experimenting with GHB might not fully comprehend the risk of addiction.

Depression and Respiratory Depression:

GHB's depressant effects can lead to depressive symptoms and mood changes, which might exacerbate any existing mental health issues in adolescents.

Respiratory depression can occur, where breathing becomes dangerously slow and shallow. This can lead to oxygen deprivation and other health complications.

Interaction with Alcohol and Other Drugs:

GHB should not be used with alcohol or other depressant drugs due to the heightened risk of respiratory depression, overdose, and other adverse effects.

Legal Consequences:

GHB is considered a controlled substance and is illegal to possess or use without a prescription. Adolescents caught using GHB can face legal repercussions.

Lack of Regulation:

GHB obtained illegally is often produced in unregulated settings, leading to inconsistent potency and quality, which increases the risk of unpredictable reactions.

Inadequate Understanding:

Adolescents might not fully understand the potential dangers of GHB, particularly if they are unaware of its depressant effects and potential for overdose.

Preventing GHB use among children and teenagers requires education, open communication, and creating supportive environments. Parents, schools, and community organizations play vital roles in raising awareness about the risks associated with GHB and other substances. It's important to encourage healthy coping mechanisms, emotional resilience, and responsible decision-making to protect young individuals from the potential dangers of GHB use.

Chapter 10 – Hallucinogens

Hallucinogens are a class of drugs that alter perception, thoughts, and feelings, often causing hallucinations or profound alterations in sensory experiences. Using hallucinogens can be especially risky for children and teenagers due to their developing brains and emotional vulnerabilities. Here are some of the key dangers associated with hallucinogen use among this age group:

Psychological Effects:

Hallucinogens can induce intense and unpredictable psychological effects, including hallucinations, altered perceptions of time and space, and distorted thoughts. Adolescents might struggle to interpret these experiences, leading to confusion and anxiety.

Mental Health Risks:

Adolescents are more susceptible to the negative psychological effects of hallucinogens. Using these substances can exacerbate or trigger mental health issues such as anxiety, depression, or psychosis.

Bad Trips:

A "bad trip" refers to a negative and distressing experience while under the influence of hallucinogens. Adolescents might be less equipped to manage and navigate these experiences, which could lead to long-lasting emotional trauma.

Flashbacks:

Hallucinogen use can result in flashbacks, which are unexpected reoccurrences of the drug's effects days, weeks, or even months after use. These flashbacks can be distressing and disruptive to everyday life.

Physical Health Risks:

The use of hallucinogens can lead to physical health risks such as increased heart rate, elevated blood pressure, and impaired coordination. Adolescents' developing bodies might be more vulnerable to these effects.

Risky Behaviors:

Hallucinogen use can impair judgment and decision-making, leading to risky behaviors such as accidents, injuries, and unprotected sex.

Education and Performance:

Adolescents who use hallucinogens might experience difficulties in school, as these substances can impact cognitive functions, memory, and concentration.

Legal Consequences:

The use of many hallucinogens is illegal. Adolescents caught using these substances can face legal repercussions that might impact their future opportunities.

Lack of Understanding:

Adolescents might lack the emotional and cognitive maturity required to understand and process the effects of hallucinogens, making them more susceptible to negative outcomes.

Substance Interactions:

Hallucinogens can interact with other substances, including medications or alcohol, leading to dangerous and unpredictable reactions.

Inaccurate Dosages:

The potency of hallucinogens can vary significantly, and adolescents might be more likely to consume inaccurate dosages, leading to unintended and potentially harmful effects.

Preventing hallucinogen use among children and teenagers requires education, open communication, and supportive environments. Parents, schools, and community organizations play crucial roles in raising awareness about the risks associated with these substances and providing adolescents with accurate information. Fostering healthy coping mechanisms, positive self-esteem, and emotional resilience can also help protect young individuals from the potential dangers of hallucinogen use.

Chapter 11 – Heroin

Heroin is a highly potent and addictive opioid drug derived from morphine. Its use poses significant dangers, particularly for children and teenagers, who are more vulnerable to its effects due to their developing bodies and brains. Here are some of the key dangers associated with heroin use among this age group:

Addiction and Dependence:

Heroin is highly addictive, and adolescents who use it are at an increased risk of developing a substance use disorder, leading to physical and psychological dependence.

Health Risks:

Heroin use can lead to a range of serious health problems, including respiratory depression, heart problems, and infections such as HIV and hepatitis from sharing needles.

Overdose and Death:

Heroin use carries a significant risk of overdose, which can lead to respiratory failure, coma, and death. Adolescents' developing bodies might be more susceptible to the toxic effects of heroin.

Physical and Cognitive Impairment:

Heroin impairs motor skills, cognitive function, and decision-making. Adolescents using heroin might struggle with academic performance and other daily activities.

Mental Health Risks:

Heroin use can exacerbate or trigger mental health issues such as depression, anxiety, and even psychosis. Adolescents might be particularly vulnerable to these effects.

Financial and Legal Consequences:

Maintaining a heroin addiction can lead to financial strain due to the high cost of the drug. Adolescents might engage in illegal activities to obtain funds, leading to legal repercussions.

Risky Behaviors:

Heroin use can lead to risky behaviors such as engaging in unsafe sexual practices and driving under the influence, which can result in accidents and injuries.

Educational and Career Impact:

Heroin use can negatively impact educational attainment and limit future career opportunities due to compromised cognitive and academic abilities.

Social Isolation:

Adolescents using heroin might withdraw from healthy social relationships and activities, isolating themselves from family and peers.

Withdrawal Symptoms:

Stopping heroin use can lead to severe withdrawal symptoms, including intense cravings, nausea, vomiting, and muscle pain.

Misinformation and Peer Pressure:

Adolescents might be influenced by misinformation and peer pressure to experiment with drugs like heroin, not fully understanding the potential consequences.

Lack of Regulation:

Heroin obtained illegally is often produced and sold in unregulated environments, increasing the risk of adulteration and unpredictable potency.

Preventing heroin use among children and teenagers requires comprehensive education, open communication, and creating supportive environments. Parents, schools, and community organizations play crucial roles in raising awareness about the dangers of heroin and other substances. Encouraging healthy coping mechanisms, positive self-esteem, and emotional resilience can help protect young individuals from the potential dangers of heroin use.

Chapter 12 – Inhalants

Inhalants are volatile substances that produce chemical vapors that can be inhaled to induce a psychoactive or mind-altering effect. These substances are often household products and include items like glue, aerosol sprays, cleaning agents, and gasoline. Inhalant use, particularly among children and teenagers, can lead to serious and potentially life-threatening consequences due to the harmful effects these substances have on the brain and body. Here are some of the key dangers associated with inhalant use among this age group:

Immediate Health Risks:

Inhalants can cause immediate and intense effects, including dizziness, lightheadedness, nausea, and confusion. Adolescents might be attracted to the quick onset of these effects, not fully understanding the risks.

Brain and Nervous System Damage:

Inhalants can cause significant damage to the brain and nervous system, leading to cognitive impairments, memory problems, and difficulties with concentration and learning.

Physical Health Risks:

Inhalant use can damage various organs, including the heart, liver, kidneys, and lungs. It can also lead to irregular heartbeats, breathing difficulties, and even sudden death.

Hypoxia and Oxygen Deprivation:

Inhalants can displace oxygen in the lungs and bloodstream, leading to hypoxia (oxygen deprivation). This can result in seizures, permanent brain damage, and even death.

Sudden Sniffing Death Syndrome:

Inhaling certain substances, particularly volatile solvents, can trigger "sudden sniffing death syndrome," a condition where the heart suddenly stops beating, leading to death.

Mental Health Risks:

Inhalant use is associated with mental health issues such as depression, anxiety, and aggressive behavior. Adolescents might be more vulnerable to these effects due to their developing brains.

Injuries and Accidents:

The intoxicating effects of inhalants can impair coordination and judgment, leading to accidents, injuries, and dangerous behaviors.

Addiction Potential:

Some inhalants have addictive properties, and adolescents using these substances might be at risk of developing a substance use disorder.

Legal Consequences:

In many places, inhalant use is illegal, especially among minors. Adolescents caught using inhalants can face legal repercussions.

Misinformation and Peer Pressure:

Adolescents might experiment with inhalants due to misinformation or peer pressure, not fully comprehending the potential dangers.

Lack of Awareness:

Adolescents might not fully understand the potential risks associated with inhalant use, as these substances are often easily accessible at home.

Sensitization to Substances:

Prolonged inhalant use can lead to sensitization, where the body becomes more sensitive to the effects of other substances, potentially leading to substance abuse.

Preventing inhalant use among children and teenagers requires education, open communication, and responsible storage of household products. Parents, schools, and community organizations play crucial roles in raising awareness about the dangers of inhalant use. Fostering healthy coping mechanisms, positive self-esteem, and emotional resilience can help protect young individuals from the potential dangers of inhalant use.

Chapter 13 – Ketamine

Ketamine is a dissociative anesthetic that is used medically for certain surgical procedures and pain management. However, when used recreationally or without proper medical supervision, ketamine can pose serious dangers, especially for children and teenagers. Here are some of the key dangers associated with ketamine use among this age group:

Cognitive Impairment:

Ketamine can cause cognitive impairment, affecting memory, attention, and decision-making. Adolescents might struggle with academic performance and other cognitive tasks.

Physical Health Risks:

Ketamine can lead to physical effects such as dizziness, loss of coordination, and nausea. Adolescents' developing bodies might be more susceptible to these effects.

Psychological Effects:

Ketamine can induce hallucinations, altered perceptions, and emotional experiences. Adolescents might have difficulty processing these effects, leading to anxiety, confusion, and distress.

Mental Health Risks:

Adolescents are more susceptible to the negative psychological effects of ketamine, including anxiety, paranoia, and exacerbation of pre-existing mental health issues.

K-Hole:

High doses of ketamine can lead to a dissociative state known as the "K-hole," characterized by intense hallucinations, loss of physical sensations, and a distorted sense of time. Adolescents might be unprepared for this intense experience.

Risk of Accidents:

The disorienting and impaired motor skills caused by ketamine can increase the risk of accidents and injuries.

Addiction and Tolerance:

Repeated ketamine use can lead to physical and psychological dependence, as well as the development of tolerance, requiring higher doses to achieve the desired effects.

Legal Consequences:

Possession and use of ketamine without a valid medical prescription is illegal. Adolescents caught using this substance can face legal repercussions.

Misuse of Medication:

Adolescents might misuse ketamine that is intended for medical use, such as in veterinary or medical settings.

Lack of Understanding:

Adolescents might lack the emotional and cognitive maturity required to understand and process the effects of ketamine, making them more susceptible to negative outcomes.

Unpredictable Reactions:

The effects of ketamine can vary widely from person to person and even from one use to another, making it difficult for adolescents to predict the outcome.

Misinterpretation of Dangers:

Adolescents might underestimate the potential risks associated with ketamine, not fully comprehending its potential dangers.

Preventing ketamine use among children and teenagers requires education, open communication, and creating supportive environments. Parents, schools, and community organizations play crucial roles in raising awareness about the dangers of ketamine and other substances. Encouraging healthy coping mechanisms, positive self-esteem, and emotional resilience can help protect young individuals from the potential dangers of ketamine use.

Chapter 14 – Khat

Khat (Catha edulis) is a flowering plant native to East Africa and the Arabian Peninsula. Its leaves contain stimulant compounds that can have effects similar to those of amphetamines. While khat is traditionally used in some cultures for its stimulant properties, its use among children and teenagers can lead to serious dangers and consequences, especially when used inappropriately or excessively. Here are some of the key dangers associated with khat use among this age group:

Physical Health Risks:

Khat use can lead to physical effects such as increased heart rate, elevated blood pressure, and dehydration. Adolescents' developing bodies might be more vulnerable to these effects.

Addiction Potential:

Khat contains stimulant compounds that can be addictive. Adolescents using khat are at a heightened risk of developing a substance use disorder.

Cognitive and Academic Impact:

Khat use can lead to impaired cognitive function, affecting memory, attention, and academic performance.

Mental Health Risks:

Adolescents using khat might experience mental health issues such as anxiety, paranoia, and sleep disturbances.

Behavioral Changes:

Khat use can lead to mood swings, irritability, and unpredictable behavior, potentially straining relationships and leading to conflicts.

Educational and Social Impact:

Khat use can interfere with school attendance, participation in extracurricular activities, and social interactions.

Risk of Overuse:

Adolescents might underestimate the potential risks associated with khat and use it excessively, leading to health issues and diminished quality of life.

Legal Consequences:

Khat is illegal in some countries and regions. Adolescents caught using this substance can face legal repercussions.

Cultural and Ethical Considerations:

Khat use might conflict with cultural values or family expectations, leading to tensions within families and communities.

Misinterpretation of Dangers:

Adolescents might lack awareness about the potential dangers of khat, not fully comprehending its potential negative effects.

Cycle of Use:

Adolescents who start using khat at a young age are at a higher risk of developing a habit that can negatively impact their future.

Preventing khat use among children and teenagers requires education, open communication, and creating supportive environments. Parents, schools, and community organizations play crucial roles in raising awareness about the dangers of khat and other substances. Encouraging healthy coping mechanisms, positive self-esteem, and emotional resilience can help protect young individuals from the potential dangers of khat use.

Kratom (Mitragyna speciosa) is a tropical plant native to Southeast Asia, and its leaves contain compounds that can have opioid-like effects. While some proponents suggest that kratom can be used for various purposes, including pain relief and relaxation, its use among children and teenagers can lead to serious dangers and consequences. Kratom is not approved by the U.S. Food and Drug Administration (FDA) for any medical use, and its safety and efficacy are a subject of debate.

Here are some of the key dangers associated with kratom use among this age group:

Addiction and Dependence:

Kratom contains compounds that can lead to physical and psychological dependence, especially when used regularly or in high doses.

Physical Health Risks:

Kratom use can lead to physical effects such as nausea, vomiting, constipation, and loss of appetite. Adolescents' developing bodies might be more vulnerable to these effects.

Cognitive Impact:

Kratom use can lead to cognitive deficits, affecting memory, attention, and decision-making.

Mental Health Risks:

Adolescents using kratom are at an increased risk of developing mental health issues such as anxiety, depression, and even psychosis.

Behavioral Changes:

Kratom use can lead to mood swings, irritability, and changes in behavior that strain relationships and lead to conflicts.

Educational and Academic Impact:

Kratom use can interfere with school attendance, participation in extracurricular activities, and academic performance.

Risk of Overuse:

Adolescents might misuse kratom in an attempt to experience its euphoric effects, leading to health issues and diminished quality of life.

Unknown Long-Term Effects:

The long-term effects of kratom use, especially during adolescence, are not well understood. The developing brain might be particularly susceptible to harm.

Lack of Regulation:

Kratom is not regulated by the FDA, which means there is a lack of standardized dosing and quality control. This can increase the risks associated with its use.

Legal Consequences:

Kratom's legal status varies by location. Adolescents caught using kratom where it's prohibited can face legal repercussions.

Misinterpretation of Dangers:

Adolescents might lack awareness about the potential risks associated with kratom, not fully comprehending its potential negative effects.

Cycle of Use:

Adolescents who start using kratom at a young age are at a higher risk of developing a habit that can negatively impact their future.

Preventing kratom use among children and teenagers requires education, open communication, and creating supportive environments. Parents, schools, and community organizations play crucial roles in raising awareness about the dangers of kratom and other substances. Encouraging healthy coping mechanisms, positive self-esteem, and emotional resilience can help protect young individuals from the potential dangers of kratom use.

Chapter 16 - LSD (Acid)

LSD, also known as acid, is a potent hallucinogenic substance that can have profound and unpredictable effects on perception, emotions, and cognition. Its use among children and teenagers can lead to serious dangers and consequences due to their developing bodies and minds. Here are some of the key dangers associated with LSD (acid) use among this age group:

Psychological Effects:

LSD use can induce intense and often overwhelming hallucinations, altered perceptions of reality, and emotional experiences. Adolescents might struggle to process these effects, leading to anxiety, confusion, and distress.

Mental Health Risks:

Adolescents are more susceptible to the negative psychological effects of LSD, including anxiety, paranoia, and exacerbation of pre-existing mental health issues.

Risk of Bad Trips:

Adolescents might experience "bad trips" characterized by extreme fear, panic, and paranoia. These experiences can have lasting psychological effects.

Flashbacks:

LSD use can lead to "flashbacks," where individuals experience hallucinogenic effects unexpectedly, even after the drug's initial use. These flashbacks can be distressing and disruptive.

Impaired Judgment:

The altered state of consciousness induced by LSD can impair judgment and decision-making, leading to risky behaviors and accidents.

Physical Health Risks:

LSD use can lead to physical effects such as increased heart rate, high blood pressure, and loss of coordination.

Educational and Academic Impact:

LSD use can lead to cognitive deficits that affect academic performance, concentration, and memory.

Legal Consequences:

Possession and use of LSD are illegal in most places. Adolescents caught using this substance can face serious legal repercussions.

Lack of Understanding:

Adolescents might lack the emotional and cognitive maturity required to understand and process the effects of LSD, making them more susceptible to negative outcomes.

Misinterpretation of Dangers:

Adolescents might underestimate the potential risks associated with LSD use, not fully comprehending its potential dangers.

Cultural and Ethical Considerations:

LSD use might conflict with cultural values or family expectations, leading to tensions within families and communities.

Cycle of Use:

Adolescents who start using LSD at a young age are at a higher risk of becoming trapped in a cycle of substance use that can negatively impact their future.

Preventing LSD (acid) use among children and teenagers requires education, open communication, and creating supportive environments. Parents, schools, and community organizations play crucial roles in raising awareness about the dangers of LSD and other substances. Encouraging healthy coping mechanisms, positive self-esteem, and emotional resilience can help protect young individuals from the potential dangers of LSD use.

Chapter 17 - MDMA (Ecstasy/Molly)

MDMA, commonly known as Ecstasy or Molly, is a synthetic drug that produces stimulant and hallucinogenic effects. Its use among children and teenagers can lead to serious dangers and consequences due to their developing bodies and minds.

Here are some of the key dangers associated with MDMA use among this age group:

Physical Health Risks:

MDMA can lead to physical effects such as increased heart rate, high blood pressure, dehydration, and hyperthermia (dangerously elevated body temperature). Adolescents' developing bodies might be more susceptible to these effects.

Overheating and Hydration Issues:

MDMA can impair the body's ability to regulate temperature and can lead to severe overheating, which can be life-threatening, especially during crowded events like parties or concerts.

Mental Health Risks:

Adolescents are more vulnerable to the negative psychological effects of MDMA, including anxiety, depression, and emotional instability.

Memory Impairment:

MDMA use can lead to memory deficits and cognitive impairments that affect academic performance and daily functioning.

Serotonin Syndrome:

MDMA use can lead to serotonin syndrome, a potentially life-threatening condition characterized by symptoms such as agitation, confusion, high heart rate, and increased body temperature.

Behavioral Changes:

Adolescents might experience mood swings, impulsivity, and emotional instability as a result of MDMA use.

Risk of Accidents:

The impaired judgment and motor skills caused by MDMA can increase the risk of accidents and injuries.

Educational and Academic Impact:

MDMA use can lead to cognitive deficits that affect academic performance, concentration, and memory.

Legal Consequences:

Possession and use of MDMA are illegal in most places. Adolescents caught using this substance can face serious legal repercussions.

Lack of Understanding:

Adolescents might lack the emotional and cognitive maturity required to understand and process the effects of MDMA, making them more susceptible to negative outcomes.

Misinterpretation of Dangers:

Adolescents might underestimate the potential risks associated with MDMA use, not fully comprehending its potential dangers.

Cycle of Use:

Adolescents who start using MDMA at a young age are at a higher risk of becoming trapped in a cycle of substance use that can negatively impact their future.

Preventing MDMA (Ecstasy/Molly) use among children and teenagers requires education, open communication, and creating supportive environments. Parents, schools, and community organizations play crucial roles in raising awareness about the dangers of MDMA and other substances. Encouraging healthy coping mechanisms, positive self-esteem, and emotional resilience can help protect young individuals from the potential dangers of MDMA use.

Chapter 18 - Mescaline (Peyote)

Mescaline is a naturally occurring psychedelic compound found in certain cacti, most notably in the Peyote cactus. While mescaline has been used for centuries in religious and cultural contexts, its use among children and teenagers can lead to serious dangers and consequences due to their developing bodies and minds. Here are some of the key dangers associated with mescaline (Peyote) use among this age group:

Psychological Effects:

Mescaline use can lead to intense and often unpredictable hallucinations, altered perceptions of reality, and emotional experiences. Adolescents might struggle to process these effects, leading to anxiety, confusion, and distress.

Mental Health Risks:

Adolescents are more susceptible to the negative psychological effects of mescaline, including anxiety, paranoia, and exacerbation of pre-existing mental health issues.

Cognitive Impairment:

Mescaline use can impair cognitive function, affecting memory, attention, and decision-making.

Risk of Bad Trips:

Adolescents might experience "bad trips" characterized by overwhelming fear, paranoia, and panic. These experiences can have long-lasting psychological effects.

Physical Health Risks:

Mescaline use can lead to physical effects such as nausea, vomiting, increased heart rate, and high blood pressure.

Accidental Ingestion:

Mescaline can be toxic in high doses. Adolescents might be at risk of accidental overdose due to the variability in potency of the substance.

Educational and Academic Impact:

Mescaline use can lead to cognitive deficits that affect academic performance, concentration, and memory.

Lack of Understanding:

Adolescents might lack the emotional and cognitive maturity required to understand and process the effects of mescaline, making them more susceptible to negative outcomes.

Legal Consequences:

Possession and use of mescaline-containing substances might be illegal in some places. Adolescents caught using these substances can face legal repercussions.

Misinterpretation of Dangers:

Adolescents might underestimate the potential risks associated with mescaline use, not fully comprehending its potential dangers.

Cultural and Ethical Considerations:

Mescaline use might conflict with cultural values or family expectations, leading to tensions within families and communities.

Cycle of Use:

Adolescents who start using mescaline at a young age are at a higher risk of becoming trapped in a cycle of substance use that can negatively impact their future.

Preventing mescaline (Peyote) use among children and teenagers requires education, open communication, and creating supportive environments. Parents, schools, and community organizations play crucial roles in raising awareness about the dangers of mescaline and other substances. Encouraging healthy coping mechanisms, positive self-esteem, and emotional resilience can help protect young individuals from the potential dangers of mescaline use.

Chapter 19 - Methamphetamine (Crystal/Meth)

Methamphetamine, commonly known as crystal meth or meth, is a highly addictive and potent stimulant that can have severe and lasting effects on the physical, mental, and social well-being of children and teenagers. The use of methamphetamine among this age group can lead to serious dangers and consequences due to their developing bodies and brains. Here are some of the key dangers associated with methamphetamine use among children and teenagers:

Addiction and Dependence:

Methamphetamine is highly addictive, and adolescents using this drug are at a heightened risk of developing a substance use disorder.

Physical Health Risks:

Methamphetamine can lead to physical effects such as increased heart rate, high blood pressure, dental problems (often referred to as "meth mouth"), weight loss, and skin sores.

Neurological and Cognitive Impact:

Methamphetamine can cause damage to brain cells and lead to cognitive deficits, memory problems, and difficulties with attention and decision-making. Adolescents' developing brains might be more vulnerable to these effects.

Mental Health Risks:

Adolescents using methamphetamine are at an increased risk of developing mental health issues such as anxiety, paranoia, aggression, and even psychosis.

Behavioral Changes:

Methamphetamine use can lead to erratic and aggressive behavior, increasing the risk of accidents, injuries, and interpersonal conflicts.

Educational and Academic Impact:

Methamphetamine use can lead to impaired cognitive function, affecting academic performance, concentration, and memory.

Social Isolation:

Adolescents using methamphetamine might isolate themselves from healthy social interactions, leading to strained relationships and social isolation.

Legal Consequences:

Possession and use of methamphetamine are illegal in most places. Adolescents caught using this substance can face serious legal repercussions.

Risk of Overdose:

Methamphetamine overdose can lead to seizures, stroke, heart attack, and even death. Adolescents might be more vulnerable to these risks due to their developing bodies.

Misinterpretation of Dangers:

Adolescents might underestimate the potential risks associated with methamphetamine, not fully comprehending its potential dangers.

Cycle of Addiction:

Adolescents who start using methamphetamine at a young age are at a higher risk of becoming trapped in a cycle of addiction that can have lasting negative effects on their lives.

Preventing methamphetamine use among children and teenagers requires education, open communication, and creating supportive environments. Parents, schools, and community organizations play crucial roles in raising awareness about the dangers of methamphetamine and other substances. Encouraging healthy coping mechanisms, positive self-esteem, and emotional resilience can help protect young individuals from the potential dangers of methamphetamine use.

Chapter 20 - Over-the-Counter Medicines—Dextromethorphan (DXM)

Dextromethorphan (DXM) is a common active ingredient found in many over-the-counter cough and cold medications. When used as directed, it can provide relief from coughing. However, misuse or abuse of DXM, particularly by children and teenagers, can lead to serious health risks and consequences. DXM is often abused for its dissociative and hallucinogenic effects. Here are some of the key dangers associated with DXM use among this age group:

Psychological Effects:

DXM misuse can lead to intense dissociation, hallucinations, and altered perceptions of reality. Adolescents might struggle to process these effects, leading to confusion, anxiety, and emotional distress.

Mental Health Risks:

Adolescents are more susceptible to the negative psychological effects of DXM, including anxiety, paranoia, and exacerbation of pre-existing mental health issues.

Physical Health Risks:

Misusing DXM can lead to physical effects such as dizziness, increased heart rate, and impaired coordination. Adolescents' developing bodies might be more vulnerable to these effects.

Risk of Accidents:

The disorienting and impaired motor skills caused by DXM can increase the risk of accidents and injuries.

Addiction Potential:

Adolescents misusing DXM might develop a pattern of misuse due to its potential to produce euphoria and altered states of consciousness.

Serotonin Syndrome:

DXM misuse can lead to serotonin syndrome when combined with other substances that affect serotonin levels, potentially resulting in severe and life-threatening symptoms.

Cognitive Impairment:

Misusing DXM can lead to cognitive impairment, affecting memory, attention, and decision-making.

Interaction with Other Medications:

DXM can interact with other medications or substances, leading to dangerous side effects or unpredictable reactions.

Educational and Academic Impact:

DXM misuse can lead to cognitive deficits, impacting academic performance, concentration, and memory.

Lack of Understanding:

Adolescents might not fully understand the potential risks associated with DXM misuse, perceiving it as a harmless over-the-counter medication.

Misuse of Trust:

Adolescents might misuse DXM in an attempt to experience dissociation or hallucinations, potentially leading to harm and loss of trust.

Legal Consequences:

While DXM is available over the counter, its misuse can still have legal consequences, especially if taken in excessive amounts or in a manner not intended by the manufacturer.

Preventing DXM misuse among children and teenagers requires education, open communication, and creating supportive environments. Parents, schools, and community organizations play crucial roles in raising awareness about the dangers of misusing over-the-counter medications. Encouraging healthy habits, responsible medication use, and emotional resilience can help protect young individuals from the potential dangers of DXM misuse.

Chapter 21 - Over-the-Counter Medicines—Loperamide

Loperamide is an over-the-counter medication commonly used to treat diarrhea. When taken as directed, it is generally safe and effective. However, misuse or abuse of loperamide, particularly by children and teenagers, can lead to serious health risks and consequences. Here are some of the key dangers associated with loperamide use among this age group:

Cardiac Effects:

High doses of loperamide can lead to cardiac toxicity, including dangerous changes in heart rhythm. Adolescents might be more susceptible to these effects due to their developing cardiovascular systems.

Respiratory Depression:

Misuse of loperamide can lead to respiratory depression, where breathing becomes slow and shallow. This can be especially risky for adolescents with developing respiratory systems.

Central Nervous System Effects:

Loperamide misuse can cause central nervous system depression, leading to drowsiness, confusion, and impaired coordination.

Gastrointestinal Distress:

Taking excessive doses of loperamide can lead to severe gastrointestinal distress, including constipation, bloating, and abdominal pain.

Kidney and Liver Damage:

Misuse of loperamide can potentially cause damage to the kidneys and liver, especially with prolonged or excessive use.

Addiction Potential:

Adolescents misusing loperamide might develop a pattern of misuse due to its potential to produce opioid-like effects.

Interaction with Other Medications:

Loperamide can interact with other medications, leading to dangerous side effects or reduced effectiveness of other treatments.

Misuse of Trust:

Adolescents might misuse loperamide in an attempt to experience opioid-like effects, potentially leading to harm and loss of trust.

Educational and Academic Impact:

Misusing loperamide can lead to cognitive impairment and affect academic performance, concentration, and memory.

Legal Consequences:

While loperamide is available over the counter, its misuse can still have legal consequences, especially if taken in excessive amounts or in a manner not intended by the manufacturer.

Lack of Understanding:

Adolescents might not fully understand the potential risks associated with loperamide misuse, perceiving it as a harmless over-the-counter medication.

Unregulated Use:

Misuse of loperamide obtained over the counter might not be accurately dosed, leading to unpredictable and potentially harmful effects.

Preventing loperamide misuse among children and teenagers requires education, open communication, and creating supportive environments. Parents, schools, and community organizations play crucial roles in raising awareness about the dangers of misusing over-the-counter medications. Encouraging healthy habits, responsible medication use, and emotional resilience can help protect young individuals from the potential dangers of loperamide misuse.

Chapter 22 - PCP (Angel Dust)

Phencyclidine (PCP), commonly known as "angel dust," is a powerful dissociative anesthetic that was initially developed for medical use but is now illegal in many places due to its potential for abuse and serious health risks. The use of PCP among children and teenagers can lead to severe dangers and consequences, particularly due to their developing bodies and brains. Here are some of the key dangers associated with PCP use among this age group:

Psychological Effects:

PCP can induce intense hallucinations, distorted perceptions of reality, and emotional instability. Adolescents might have difficulty processing these effects, leading to anxiety, confusion, and aggression.

Aggressive Behavior:

PCP use is associated with unpredictable and aggressive behavior, which can put both the user and those around them at risk.

Physical Health Risks:

PCP use can lead to physical effects such as numbness, loss of coordination, and impaired motor skills. Adolescents' developing bodies might be more vulnerable to these effects.

Injury Risk:

The disorienting and anesthetic effects of PCP can impair judgment and coordination, increasing the risk of accidents and injuries.

Mental Health Risks:

Adolescents using PCP are more susceptible to the negative psychological effects, including anxiety, paranoia, depression, and even psychosis.

Memory Impairment:

PCP can lead to memory impairment and cognitive difficulties, affecting academic performance and daily functioning.

Violent Tendencies:

The aggressive and unpredictable behavior associated with PCP use can lead to violent confrontations and dangerous situations.

Dependence and Addiction:

Repeated PCP use can lead to physical and psychological dependence, as well as addiction. Adolescents might be more susceptible to developing a substance use disorder.

Legal Consequences:

Possession and use of PCP are illegal in many places. Adolescents caught using this substance can face serious legal repercussions.

Lack of Understanding:

Adolescents might lack the emotional and cognitive maturity required to understand and process the effects of PCP, making them more susceptible to negative outcomes.

Unpredictable Reactions:

The effects of PCP can vary widely from person to person and even from one use to another, making it difficult for adolescents to anticipate the outcome.

Misinterpretation of Dangers:

Adolescents might underestimate the potential risks associated with PCP, not fully comprehending its potential dangers.

Preventing PCP use among children and teenagers requires education, open communication, and creating supportive environments. Parents, schools, and community organizations play crucial roles in raising awareness about the dangers of PCP and other substances. Encouraging healthy coping mechanisms, positive self-esteem, and emotional resilience can help protect young individuals from the potential dangers of PCP use.

Chapter 23 - Prescription Opioids (Oxy/Percs)

Prescription opioids, including medications like OxyContin and Percocet, are powerful pain relievers often prescribed by doctors for managing moderate to severe pain. However, the misuse and abuse of prescription opioids, especially by children and teenagers, can have serious health risks and consequences. Here are some of the key dangers associated with prescription opioid use among this age group:

Addiction and Dependence:

Prescription opioids are highly addictive, and adolescents who misuse or abuse them are at an increased risk of developing a substance use disorder. Early exposure to opioids can lead to long-term dependence.

Health Risks:

Misusing prescription opioids can lead to a range of health problems, including respiratory depression, heart problems, and gastrointestinal issues. Adolescents' developing bodies might be more susceptible to these effects.

Overdose and Death:

Prescription opioid misuse carries a significant risk of overdose, leading to respiratory depression, unconsciousness, and even death. Adolescents' tolerance might be lower, increasing the risk of overdose.

Mental Health Risks:

The misuse of prescription opioids can lead to mental health issues such as depression, anxiety, and mood swings. Adolescents might be particularly vulnerable to these effects.

Accidental Poisoning:

Adolescents might accidentally ingest prescription opioids that are not meant for them, which can lead to serious health risks, especially for younger children.

Risky Behaviors:

Opioid use can impair judgment and coordination, leading to risky behaviors such as accidents, injuries, and unsafe sexual practices.

Educational and Academic Impact:

Misusing prescription opioids can lead to cognitive impairment and academic difficulties, affecting school performance and future opportunities.

Gateway to Other Substances:

Misusing prescription opioids can increase the likelihood of experimenting with other substances, leading to a potentially dangerous pattern of substance abuse.

Withdrawal Symptoms:

Adolescents who misuse prescription opioids might experience withdrawal symptoms if they attempt to stop. These symptoms can be physically and mentally distressing.

Lack of Regulation:

Obtaining prescription opioids without a valid prescription can lead to the use of counterfeit or adulterated medications, increasing the risk of negative health effects.

Social Isolation:

Adolescents who misuse prescription opioids might isolate themselves from friends and family, leading to strained relationships and a lack of social support.

Misuse of Family Medications:

Adolescents might access prescription opioids from their family's medicine cabinets, potentially leading to unintended consequences for other family members.

Preventing prescription opioid misuse among children and teenagers requires education, open communication, and responsible use of these medications. Parents, healthcare providers, schools, and community organizations all play vital roles in raising awareness about the dangers of prescription opioid misuse. Encouraging healthy pain management strategies, responsible medication storage, and emotional resilience can help protect young individuals from the potential dangers of prescription opioid use.

Chapter 24 - Prescription Stimulants (Speed)

Prescription stimulants, including medications like Adderall and Ritalin, are commonly prescribed to treat conditions like attention-deficit/hyperactivity disorder (ADHD). However, when misused or abused by children and teenagers without a legitimate medical need, these substances can have serious health risks and consequences. Here are some of the key dangers associated with prescription stimulant use among this age group:

Cardiovascular Risks:

Prescription stimulants can increase heart rate, blood pressure, and the risk of heart problems. Adolescents' developing cardiovascular systems might be more susceptible to these effects.

Mental Health Risks:

Misusing prescription stimulants can lead to mental health issues such as anxiety, paranoia, aggression, and even psychosis. Adolescents might be particularly vulnerable to these effects.

Addiction and Dependence:

Prescription stimulants are potential substances of abuse, and adolescents misusing these medications are at an increased risk of developing a substance use disorder.

Cognitive and Academic Impact:

Stimulant misuse can lead to cognitive impairment, affecting memory, attention, and academic performance. Adolescents might struggle with learning and concentrating.

Physical Health Risks:

Misusing stimulants can lead to physical health issues such as insomnia, weight loss, and headaches. Adolescents might be more susceptible to these effects due to their developing bodies.

Risky Behaviors:

Stimulant use can lead to risky behaviors such as impulsivity, reckless driving, and engaging in dangerous activities.

Misuse of Medication:

Adolescents might misuse prescription stimulants to stay awake for extended periods, especially during exams or to increase productivity.

Withdrawal Symptoms:

Stopping stimulant use after a period of misuse can lead to withdrawal symptoms such as fatigue, depression, and increased appetite.

Educational and Career Impact:

Stimulant misuse can lead to academic difficulties, impact educational attainment, and limit future career opportunities due to compromised cognitive abilities.

Legal Consequences:

Misusing prescription stimulants without a prescription is illegal. Adolescents caught using these substances without medical supervision can face legal repercussions.

Peer Pressure and Academic Pressure:

Adolescents might misuse prescription stimulants due to peer pressure or academic stress, not fully understanding the potential dangers.

Lack of Regulation:

Obtaining prescription stimulants without a valid prescription can lead to the use of counterfeit or adulterated medications, increasing the risk of negative health effects.

Preventing prescription stimulant misuse among children and teenagers requires education, open communication, and responsible use of these medications. Parents, healthcare providers, schools, and community organizations all play crucial roles in raising awareness about the dangers of stimulant misuse. Encouraging healthy studying habits, stress management strategies, and emotional resilience can help

protect young individuals from the potential dangers of
prescription stimulant use.

Chapter 25 - Psilocybin (Magic Mushrooms/Shrooms)

Psilocybin, commonly referred to as magic mushrooms or shrooms, is a naturally occurring hallucinogenic compound found in certain types of mushrooms. The use of psilocybin among children and teenagers can pose serious risks and dangers due to their developing brains and emotional vulnerabilities. Here are some of the key dangers associated with psilocybin use among this age group:

Psychological Effects:

Psilocybin can induce intense hallucinations, altered perceptions, and emotional experiences. Adolescents might struggle to process these effects, leading to confusion, anxiety, and emotional distress.

Mental Health Risks:

Adolescents are more susceptible to the negative psychological effects of psilocybin, including anxiety, panic attacks, and even exacerbation of existing mental health issues.

Bad Trips:

A "bad trip" refers to a negative and distressing experience while under the influence of psilocybin. Adolescents might be less equipped to manage and navigate these experiences, which could lead to long-lasting emotional trauma.

Flashbacks:

Psilocybin use can result in flashbacks, where individuals experience hallucinogenic effects unexpectedly, even after the drug's initial use. These flashbacks can be distressing and disruptive.

Physical Health Risks:

The use of psilocybin can lead to physical health risks such as nausea, vomiting, increased heart rate, and impaired coordination. Adolescents' developing bodies might be more vulnerable to these effects.

Lack of Understanding:

Adolescents might lack the emotional and cognitive maturity required to understand and process the effects of psilocybin, making them more susceptible to negative outcomes.

Legal Consequences:

The use of psilocybin-containing mushrooms is illegal in many places, including for minors. Adolescents caught using these substances can face legal repercussions.

Educational and Academic Impact:

Psilocybin use can lead to difficulties in school and impair cognitive function, memory, and concentration.

Social and Interpersonal Impact:

Adolescents who use psilocybin might isolate themselves from healthy social interactions, leading to strained relationships and potential social isolation.

Misinformation and Peer Pressure:

Adolescents might be influenced by misinformation or peer pressure to experiment with substances like psilocybin, not fully understanding the potential dangers.

Misinterpretation of Dangers:

Adolescents might underestimate the potential risks associated with psilocybin, perceiving it as a harmless or natural substance.

Interactions with Other Substances:

Psilocybin can interact with other substances, leading to unpredictable and potentially dangerous reactions.

Preventing psilocybin use among children and teenagers requires education, open communication, and creating supportive environments. Parents, schools, and community organizations play crucial roles in raising awareness about the potential dangers of psilocybin and other substances. Fostering healthy coping mechanisms, positive self-esteem, and emotional resilience can help protect young individuals from the potential dangers of psilocybin use.

Chapter 26 - Rohypnol®
(Flunitrazepam/Roofies)

Rohypnol® (generic name: flunitrazepam) is a powerful sedative and hypnotic drug that is not approved for medical use in the United States but is available in some other countries. It has gained notoriety as a "date rape drug" due to its ability to incapacitate individuals and impair memory and judgment. The misuse of Rohypnol, especially by children and teenagers, can have severe and potentially life-threatening consequences. Here are some of the key dangers associated with Rohypnol use among this age group:

Impaired Judgment and Memory:

Rohypnol can cause memory loss, confusion, and impaired judgment. Adolescents who use this drug might engage in risky behaviors or put themselves in dangerous situations without realizing it.

Sexual Assault and Date Rape:

Rohypnol is notorious for its potential use in facilitating sexual assault and date rape. Adolescents who unknowingly consume Rohypnol might become vulnerable to sexual exploitation and manipulation.

Physical and Psychological Effects:

Rohypnol can cause physical effects such as drowsiness, dizziness, and muscle relaxation. Adolescents might struggle to recognize and respond to these effects appropriately.

Respiratory Depression:

Rohypnol, like other central nervous system depressants, can lead to respiratory depression, which can be especially dangerous in adolescents due to their developing respiratory systems.

Unpredictable Reactions:

The effects of Rohypnol can vary widely from person to person, making it difficult for adolescents to predict how the drug will affect them.

Memory Blackouts:

Adolescents using Rohypnol might experience memory blackouts and have difficulty remembering events that occurred while under its influence.

Addiction Potential:

Repeated misuse of Rohypnol can lead to physical and psychological dependence, potentially setting the stage for a long-term substance use disorder.

Misuse of Trust:

Adolescents might be more vulnerable to being offered Rohypnol by acquaintances, peers, or even friends, leading to a breach of trust and potential harm.

Legal Consequences:

Possession and use of Rohypnol without a valid prescription is illegal. Adolescents caught using this substance can face legal repercussions.

Lack of Awareness:

Adolescents might not be adequately aware of the risks associated with Rohypnol and might not recognize its presence in their environment.

GHB and Alcohol Interaction:

Combining Rohypnol with other substances, especially alcohol or GHB, can lead to dangerous interactions and increased risk of adverse effects.

Preventing the misuse of Rohypnol among children and teenagers requires education, open communication, and creating supportive environments. Parents, schools, and community organizations play vital roles in raising awareness about the dangers of this substance and other date rape drugs. It's essential to encourage healthy boundaries, safe social behaviors, and awareness of personal safety to protect young individuals from the potential dangers of Rohypnol use.

Chapter 27 – Salvia

Salvia divinorum, commonly known as salvia, is a potent hallucinogenic plant that has gained popularity as a recreational drug. The use of salvia among children and teenagers can lead to serious risks and dangers due to the unpredictable and powerful effects of the substance. Here are some of the key dangers associated with salvia use among this age group:

Intense Hallucinations:

Salvia can induce intense and often disturbing hallucinations and altered perceptions of reality. Adolescents might have difficulty processing these effects, leading to confusion, anxiety, and distress.

Mental Health Risks:

Adolescents are more susceptible to the negative psychological effects of salvia, including anxiety, paranoia, and panic attacks. Those with a predisposition to mental health issues might experience exacerbated symptoms.

Injury Risk:

The disorienting effects of salvia can impair motor skills and coordination, increasing the risk of accidents and injuries.

Physical Health Risks:

Salvia can lead to physical effects such as dizziness, loss of balance, and nausea. Adolescents' developing bodies might be more susceptible to these effects.

Flashbacks:

The use of salvia can lead to flashbacks, where individuals experience hallucinogenic effects unexpectedly, even after the drug's initial use. These flashbacks can be distressing and disruptive.

Lack of Control:

Adolescents might struggle to control or regulate their experiences while under the influence of salvia, leading to a sense of helplessness and vulnerability.

Risk of Accidents:

The dissociative effects of salvia can lead to accidents and injuries, especially if adolescents attempt to move or navigate while experiencing altered perceptions.

Misinterpretation of Reality:

Adolescents might have difficulty distinguishing between the hallucinogenic experience and reality, leading to confusion and potential distress.

Misuse of Trust:

Adolescents might be more vulnerable to experimentation with salvia offered by peers, leading to potential harm and loss of trust.

Legal Consequences:

In many places, the use and possession of salvia are either restricted or illegal. Adolescents caught using this substance can face legal repercussions.

Unpredictable Reactions:

The effects of salvia can vary widely from person to person and even from one use to another, making it difficult for adolescents to anticipate the outcome.

Preventing salvia use among children and teenagers requires education, open communication, and creating supportive environments. Parents, schools, and community organizations play crucial roles in raising awareness about the dangers of salvia and other hallucinogenic substances. Encouraging healthy coping mechanisms, positive self-esteem, and emotional resilience can help protect young individuals from the potential dangers of salvia use.

Chapter 28 - Steroids (Anabolic)

Anabolic steroids are synthetic variations of the male sex hormone testosterone. They are often used illegally to enhance muscle growth, physical performance, and appearance. However, anabolic steroid use among children and teenagers poses serious health risks and potential long-term consequences. Here are some of the key dangers associated with anabolic steroid use among this age group:

Stunted Growth and Development:

Adolescence is a critical period for growth and development. Anabolic steroids can prematurely close the growth plates in bones, leading to stunted height and potential long-term effects on overall physical development.

Hormonal Imbalances:

Steroid use can disrupt the normal hormonal balance in the body, leading to a range of negative effects. This includes reduced production of natural testosterone, which can lead to sexual and reproductive health issues.

Cardiovascular Risks:

Anabolic steroids can increase the risk of heart problems such as high blood pressure, heart attacks, and strokes, particularly in young individuals whose cardiovascular systems are still developing.

Liver Damage:

The use of oral anabolic steroids can strain the liver, potentially leading to liver damage or dysfunction. Young individuals might be more vulnerable to these effects due to their developing bodies.

Mental Health Risks:

Anabolic steroid use has been linked to mood swings, aggression, irritability, and even mental health disorders like depression and anxiety, especially in adolescents who are already vulnerable to emotional changes.

Physical Health Issues:

Steroid use can lead to a range of physical health problems such as acne, hair loss, oily skin, and the development of breasts (gynecomastia) in males. These effects can have significant impacts on self-esteem and body image.

Addiction Potential:

Steroid use can lead to psychological dependence, where individuals feel compelled to continue using the substances to maintain their desired physical appearance or performance levels.

Legal Consequences:

The non-medical use of anabolic steroids is illegal in many countries, including the United States. Adolescents caught using or possessing these substances can face legal consequences.

Misleading Expectations:

Anabolic steroids might give users the false impression that they can achieve unrealistic body ideals without putting in the necessary effort through proper nutrition, exercise, and healthy lifestyle choices.

Educational and Career Impact:

The focus on appearance and performance through steroid use might divert young individuals from their educational and career goals, limiting their potential in the long run.

Preventing anabolic steroid use among children and teenagers requires comprehensive education, awareness, and supportive environments. Open communication with young individuals about the dangers of steroid use, fostering a healthy body image, and promoting the benefits of natural and safe approaches to fitness and physical development are essential steps. Schools, healthcare professionals, and parents all play important roles in raising awareness and providing guidance to adolescents about the potential risks associated with anabolic steroids.

Chapter 29 - Synthetic Cannabinoids (K2/Spice)

Synthetic cannabinoids, often referred to as "K2" or "Spice," are human-made substances designed to mimic the effects of natural cannabinoids found in cannabis. These substances are created by spraying synthetic chemicals onto plant material that is then smoked or vaporized. While marketed as a legal alternative to cannabis, synthetic cannabinoids are associated with a wide range of dangers, especially for children and teenagers. Here are some of the key dangers associated with synthetic cannabinoids use among this age group:

Unpredictable Effects:

Synthetic cannabinoids are known for their unpredictable and highly variable effects. Users cannot reliably anticipate the type or intensity of the experience they will have, increasing the risk of adverse reactions.

Health Risks:

Physical Health Effects: Synthetic cannabinoids can lead to a range of physical health issues, including rapid heart rate, high blood pressure, nausea, vomiting, and respiratory problems. Young individuals might be more vulnerable to these effects due to their developing bodies.

Mental Health Risks:

Psychosis and Anxiety: Synthetic cannabinoids can induce severe anxiety, paranoia, hallucinations, and even psychotic episodes. Adolescents may be at a higher risk of these effects due to their developing brains.

Addiction Potential:

Rapid Onset of Addiction: The synthetic chemicals in these substances can lead to rapid addiction, especially among young users who might be more prone to risk-taking behaviors.

Behavioral and Legal Consequences:

Erratic Behavior: Synthetic cannabinoids can cause extreme agitation, aggressive behavior, and impaired judgment. Adolescents using these substances may engage in dangerous or illegal activities.

Overdose and Death:

Risk of Overdose: Synthetic cannabinoids can lead to overdose, resulting in seizures, heart problems, and even death. Adolescents' developing bodies might be more susceptible to the toxic effects of these substances.

Lack of Regulation:

Unknown Composition: Synthetic cannabinoids are often produced in unregulated environments, leading to inconsistencies in potency and composition. Users cannot be sure of what they are consuming, increasing the risk of adverse effects.

Peer Pressure and Experimentation:

Peer Influence: Adolescents are susceptible to peer pressure and might experiment with substances like synthetic cannabinoids to fit in with certain social groups or to appear more "mature."

Mimicking Cannabis:

Misrepresentation: Synthetic cannabinoids are often marketed as a legal alternative to cannabis, leading some young individuals to believe they are using a safer substance.

Long-Term Health Implications:

Cognitive Impact: Synthetic cannabinoids can have lasting effects on cognitive functions, attention, memory, and learning abilities in adolescents.

Legal Consequences:

Illegality: Synthetic cannabinoids are often classified as controlled substances due to their dangerous effects. Adolescents using these substances can face legal repercussions.

Preventing synthetic cannabinoids use among children and teenagers requires comprehensive efforts, including education, communication, and access to appropriate resources. Parents and guardians should engage in open conversations about the dangers of these substances, fostering an environment where young individuals feel comfortable seeking guidance. Schools, healthcare professionals, and community organizations play crucial roles in raising awareness and providing support to adolescents who may be at risk of using synthetic cannabinoids.

Chapter 30 - Synthetic Cathinones (Bath Salts/Flakka)

Synthetic cathinones, commonly known as "bath salts" or "flakka," are a group of synthetic drugs that can have dangerous and unpredictable effects on users, including children and teenagers. These substances are chemically designed to mimic the effects of stimulant drugs like amphetamines and ecstasy. However, they often come with a range of serious physical, mental, and behavioral risks. Here are some of the key dangers associated with synthetic cathinones use among children and teenagers:

Unpredictable Effects:

Synthetic cathinones are often produced in clandestine labs with varying compositions, making it difficult to determine their potency and effects. This unpredictability increases the risk of adverse reactions.

Health Risks:

Physical Health Effects: Synthetic cathinones can cause a range of physical health issues, including increased heart rate, high blood pressure, dehydration, and hyperthermia (elevated body temperature). These effects can be particularly harmful for young individuals.

Mental Health Risks:

Psychosis: Synthetic cathinones use can lead to severe agitation, paranoia, hallucinations, and even psychosis. Adolescents may be especially vulnerable to these mental health effects due to their developing brains.

Addiction Potential:

Rapid Onset of Addiction: The powerful and euphoric effects of synthetic cathinones can lead to rapid addiction, especially among young users who may be more impulsive and prone to risk-taking behaviors.

Behavioral and Legal Consequences:

Erratic Behavior: Synthetic cathinones can lead to extreme agitation, aggressive behavior, and impulsivity. These effects can result in dangerous situations, injuries, or legal issues.

Overdose and Death:

Risk of Overdose: Synthetic cathinones can cause overdose, leading to seizures, cardiac arrest, and death. Adolescents' developing bodies might be more susceptible to the toxic effects of these substances.

Lack of Awareness:

Lack of Information: Many young individuals might be unaware of the dangers associated with synthetic cathinones, as these substances are often misrepresented and marketed as harmless products.

Peer Pressure and Experimentation:

Peer Influence: Adolescents are particularly susceptible to peer pressure and might experiment with drugs like synthetic cathinones to fit in with certain social groups or to appear more "adult."

Mimicking Street Drugs:

Misrepresentation: Synthetic cathinones might be sold as something else, such as MDMA (ecstasy) or other street drugs. Young users might unknowingly consume these dangerous substances.

Long-Term Health Implications:

Cognitive Impact: Synthetic cathinones' impact on brain development and cognitive function in adolescents can be particularly concerning, potentially affecting memory, attention, and learning abilities.

Preventing synthetic cathinones use among children and teenagers requires a combination of education, parental involvement, community support, and access to mental health resources. Open communication with young individuals about the risks associated with these substances, fostering an environment where they can ask questions and seek guidance, and promoting healthy coping mechanisms are crucial steps in protecting their well-being. Additionally, schools, healthcare professionals, and community organizations play a vital role in raising awareness and providing assistance to adolescents who may be at risk of using synthetic cathinones.

Chapter 31 - Tobacco/Nicotine and Vaping

Tobacco/nicotine use, including vaping, poses significant dangers to children and teenagers. The rise of e-cigarettes and vaping products has introduced new risks to this age group, leading to concerns about their health, development, and well-being. Here are some of the key dangers associated with tobacco/nicotine and vaping use among children and teenagers:

Nicotine Addiction:

Vaping and Adolescents: Vaping devices often contain high levels of nicotine, which can lead to rapid addiction, especially among adolescents whose brains are still developing. Nicotine addiction can have lasting effects and increase the risk of substance use disorders in the future.

Impact on Brain Development:

Vulnerable Period: Adolescence is a critical period for brain development, and nicotine exposure during this time can disrupt cognitive functions, attention, learning, and impulse control.

Health Risks:

Respiratory Problems: Vaping has been associated with respiratory issues, including lung inflammation and damage, which can be particularly concerning for young individuals whose lungs are still developing.

Nicotine's Impact: Nicotine can harm the cardiovascular system, increasing the risk of heart problems and contributing to elevated blood pressure.

Gateway to Other Substances:

Increased Risk: Using tobacco or nicotine products at a young age can increase the likelihood of experimenting with other substances, leading to a potentially dangerous pattern of substance abuse.

Social and Academic Consequences:

Impaired Concentration: Nicotine can impair concentration and focus, potentially affecting school performance and academic achievement.

Social Isolation: Being addicted to nicotine can lead to isolation from peers who do not use tobacco or vape products, making it harder to form healthy relationships.

Financial Burden:

Long-Term Costs: Developing a nicotine addiction can lead to significant financial burdens over time as individuals need to continually purchase tobacco or vaping products.

Marketing and Peer Pressure:

Appealing Marketing: Many vaping products are marketed in ways that appeal to young individuals, potentially influencing them to start using these products.

Peer Influence: Peer pressure can play a significant role in initiating tobacco or vaping use, as adolescents may feel pressured to fit in with their social groups.

Lack of Regulation:

Unsafe Ingredients: Vaping products can contain harmful chemicals, flavorings, and additives that may have unknown long-term health consequences. The lack of strict regulations can put young users at risk.

Legal Implications:

Age Restrictions: In many jurisdictions, the sale and use of tobacco and nicotine products are restricted to individuals above a certain age. Children and teenagers using these products may face legal consequences.

Preventing tobacco/nicotine and vaping use among children and teenagers requires a comprehensive approach involving education, regulation, and support from parents, schools, and communities. Raising awareness about the dangers of nicotine addiction, the health risks associated with tobacco and vaping products, and the negative impact on development can help deter young individuals from initiating use. Creating environments that promote healthy choices and providing access to mental health and addiction resources are essential for protecting the well-being of children and teenagers.

Chapter 32 – Prevention

What is Prevention?

Prevention, in the context of keeping children and teenagers away from using drugs, refers to a range of strategies and initiatives designed to educate, inform, and empower young individuals to make healthy choices and avoid the initiation of drug use. Prevention aims to reduce the risk factors that contribute to substance abuse while enhancing protective factors that promote overall well-being and resilience. The goal of prevention is to equip children and teenagers with the knowledge, skills, and support they need to make informed decisions about their health and avoid engaging in risky behaviors such as drug use. Effective prevention strategies often involve multiple stakeholders, including parents, schools, communities, healthcare professionals, and policymakers.

Key components of drug prevention include:

Education and Awareness:

Providing accurate and age-appropriate information about the risks and consequences of drug use helps young individuals understand the potential dangers and make informed decisions.

Life Skills Development:

Teaching life skills such as communication, decision-making, problem-solving, and stress management empowers children and teenagers to resist peer pressure and cope with challenges in healthy ways.

Building Resilience:

Enhancing protective factors like self-esteem, a sense of belonging, and healthy coping mechanisms can strengthen young individuals' ability to resist substance use.

Promotion of Positive Activities:

Encouraging participation in extracurricular activities, sports, arts, and community service provides adolescents with constructive outlets for their energy and interests.

Parental Involvement:

Engaging parents and caregivers in prevention efforts helps them communicate openly with their children, set clear expectations, and provide support.

School-Based Programs:

Schools can implement evidence-based prevention programs that address substance abuse education, social skills, and conflict resolution.

Community Engagement:

Community organizations, religious institutions, and youth clubs can create safe and supportive spaces for young individuals and offer positive role models.

Media Literacy:

Teaching children and teenagers to critically evaluate media messages related to drugs helps them understand and resist marketing tactics that promote substance use.

Policy Advocacy:

Advocating for policies that regulate access to substances and limit marketing directed at youth can help create a safer environment.

Early Intervention:

Identifying and addressing risk factors early on, such as mental health challenges or family issues, can prevent the escalation of substance use.

Prevention efforts are most effective when they involve collaboration among various sectors, use evidence-based strategies, and are tailored to the specific needs and cultural contexts of the target population. By focusing on prevention, communities can work together to create a supportive environment that encourages healthy choices and reduces the likelihood of children and teenagers experimenting with drugs in the first place.

How Does One Go About Starting A Drug Use Prevention Program for Children and Teenagers?

Starting a drug use prevention program for children and teenagers involves careful planning, coordination, and implementation. Here's a step-by-step guide to help you get started:

Assess the Need:

Research the prevalence of drug use among children and teenagers in your community. Identify risk factors (such as lack of parental involvement, peer pressure, etc.) and protective factors (such as access to positive activities, supportive adults, etc.) that could influence drug use.

Set Clear Goals and Objectives:

Define the specific outcomes you want to achieve with your prevention program. Goals could include reducing drug experimentation, increasing knowledge about the risks of drug use, and promoting healthy behaviors.

Gather Resources:

Identify the resources you'll need, including funding, educational materials, curriculum, trained facilitators, and partnerships with community organizations, schools, and healthcare providers.

Develop a Comprehensive Plan:

Create a detailed plan that outlines the program's structure, activities, timeline, and evaluation methods. Consider different approaches, such as school-based workshops, community events, and outreach initiatives.

Choose Evidence-Based Strategies:

Select prevention strategies and interventions that have been proven effective through research and evaluation. Look for programs that address risk and protective factors relevant to your community.

Tailor to the Audience:

Consider the age, cultural background, and needs of your target audience (children and teenagers). Adapt your messages and activities to resonate with them.

Engage Stakeholders:

Involve parents, schools, community organizations, local businesses, healthcare professionals, and other relevant stakeholders in the planning and implementation of the program.

Develop Educational Materials:

Create engaging and age-appropriate materials, presentations, and resources that provide accurate information about the risks of drug use and promote healthy decision-making.

Train Facilitators:

If your program involves workshops or presentations, ensure that facilitators are trained to deliver the content effectively and engage participants in meaningful discussions.

Promote the Program:

Use various communication channels to raise awareness about your program, such as social media, school newsletters, community meetings, and local events.

Implement and Evaluate:

Begin delivering the program as planned. Regularly assess the program's effectiveness through surveys, feedback from participants, and data on changes in attitudes and behaviors related to drug use.

Adapt and Improve:

Continuously review the program's outcomes and adapt it based on feedback and evaluation results. Make necessary adjustments to enhance its impact.

Build Partnerships:

Collaborate with schools, community organizations, healthcare providers, law enforcement, and local government to strengthen your program's reach and impact.

Sustain the Effort:

To ensure long-term success, establish a plan for sustaining the program beyond the initial implementation phase. This may include securing ongoing funding, training new facilitators, and maintaining community engagement.

Celebrate Achievements:

Recognize and celebrate the positive outcomes and milestones achieved by your prevention program. This can motivate participants, stakeholders, and the community to stay engaged.

Starting a drug use prevention program requires commitment, dedication, and a well-structured approach. By following these steps and working collaboratively with various stakeholders, you can create a program that empowers children and teenagers to make informed, healthy choices and reduce the likelihood of drug use.

Principles of Drug Addiction Treatment – From NIDA (National Institute on Drug Abuse)

Principles of Drug Addiction Treatment

More than three decades of scientific research show that treatment can help drug-addicted individuals stop drug use, avoid relapse and successfully recover their lives. Based on this research, 13 fundamental principles that characterize effective drug abuse treatment have been developed. These principles are detailed in NIDA's Principles of Drug Addiction Treatment: A Research-Based Guide. The guide also describes different types of science-based treatments and provides answers to commonly asked questions.

1. Addiction is a complex but treatable disease that affects brain function and behavior. Drugs alter the brain's structure and how it functions, resulting in changes that persist long after drug use has ceased. This may help explain why abusers are at risk for relapse even after long periods of abstinence.

2. No single treatment is appropriate for everyone. Matching treatment settings, interventions, and services to an individual's particular problems and needs is critical to his or her ultimate success.

3. Treatment needs to be readily available. Because drug-addicted individuals may be uncertain about entering treatment, taking advantage of available services the moment people are ready for treatment is critical. Potential patients can be lost if treatment is not immediately available or readily accessible.

4. Effective treatment attends to multiple needs of the individual, not just his or her drug abuse. To be effective, treatment must address the individual's drug abuse and any associated medical, psychological, social, vocational, and legal problems.

5. Remaining in treatment for an adequate period of time is critical. The appropriate duration for an individual depends on the type and degree of his or her problems and needs. Research indicates that most addicted individuals need at least 3 months in treatment to significantly reduce or stop their drug use and that the best outcomes occur with longer durations of treatment.

6. Counseling—individual and/or group—and other behavioral therapies are the most commonly used forms of drug abuse treatment. Behavioral therapies vary in their focus and may involve addressing a patient's motivations to change, building skills to resist drug use, replacing drug-using activities with constructive and rewarding activities, improving problemsolving skills, and facilitating better interpersonal relationships.

7. Medications are an important element of treatment for many patients, especially when combined with counseling and other behavioral therapies. For example, methadone and buprenorphine are effective in helping individuals addicted to heroin or other opioids stabilize their lives and reduce their illicit drug use. Also, for persons addicted to nicotine, a nicotine replacement product (nicotine patches or gum) or an oral medication (buproprion or varenicline), can be an effective component of treatment when part of a comprehensive behavioral treatment program.

8. An individual's treatment and services plan must be assessed continually and modified as necessary to ensure it meets his or her changing needs. A patient may require varying

combinations of services and treatment components during the course of treatment and recovery. In addition to counseling or psychotherapy, a patient may require medication, medical services, family therapy, parenting instruction, vocational rehabilitation and/or social and legal services. For many patients, a continuing care approach provides the best results, with treatment intensity varying according to a person's changing needs.

9. Many drug-addicted individuals also have other mental disorders. Because drug abuse and addiction—both of which are mental disorders—often co-occur with other mental illnesses, patients presenting with one condition should be assessed for the other(s). And when these problems co-occur, treatment should address both (or all), including the use of medications as appropriate.

10. Medically assisted detoxification is only the first stage of addiction treatment and by itself does little to change long-term drug abuse. Although medically assisted detoxification can safely manage the acute physical symptoms of withdrawal, detoxification alone is rarely sufficient to help addicted individuals achieve long-term abstinence. Thus, patients should be encouraged to continue drug treatment following detoxification.

11. Treatment does not need to be voluntary to be effective. Sanctions or enticements from family, employment settings, and/or the criminal justice system can significantly increase treatment entry, retention rates, and the ultimate success of drug treatment interventions.

12. Drug use during treatment must be monitored continuously, as lapses during treatment do occur. Knowing their drug use is being monitored can be a powerful incentive for patients and can help them withstand urges to use drugs. Monitoring also

provides an early indication of a return to drug use, signaling a possible need to adjust an individual's treatment plan to better meet his or her needs.

13. Treatment programs should assess patients for the presence of HIV/AIDS, hepatitis B and C, tuberculosis, and other infectious diseases, as well as provide targeted risk-reduction counseling to help patients modify or change behaviors that place them at risk of contracting or spreading infectious diseases. Targeted counseling specifically focused on reducing infectious disease risk can help patients further reduce or avoid substance-related and other high-risk behaviors. Treatment providers should encourage and support HIV screening and inform patients that highly active antiretroviral therapy (HAART) has proven effective in combating HIV, including among drug-abusing populations.

INDEX OF SUPPORT MATERIALS

Drug Slang Code Words – Find on DEA.GOV

Nar-Anon

https://www.nar-anon.org/

"The Nar-Anon Family Groups is primarily for those who know or have known a feeling of desperation concerning the addiction problem of someone very near to you. We have traveled that unhappy road too, and found the answer with serenity and peace of mind. Narateen is part of the Nar-Anon program for teens affected by someone else's addiction."

Al-Anon Family Groups

https://al-anon.org/

Al-Anon members are people, just like you, who are worried about someone with a drinking problem.

How to find a Social Worker

https://www.helpstartshere.org/find-a-social-worker/

Social Workers can provide you with reasonably priced or free resources.